**winner
michigan writers cooperative press
2023 creative nonfiction contest**

Twinkies
Kathleen Quigley

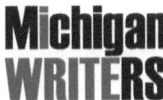

Copyright © 2023 by Kathleen Quigley. All rights reserved.

Michigan Writers Cooperative Press
P. O. Box 2355
Traverse City, Michigan 49685

ISBN-13: 978-1-950744-11-4

Book cover by Amy Hansen
Book interior by Daniel Stewart

TWINKIES

For Patty

I MET PATTY DURING A WEEKEND ORIENTATION FOR THE college we had both chosen. I suggested skinny-dipping in the fieldhouse pool; Patty thought I was wild, and I thought she was mousy. We met again at a track team meeting the first week of school and became instant best friends the way girls do in college.

At a party one night she said, "I'm going to die young."

"You're full of shit. What makes you think that?"

"I can't imagine being twenty-five or older."

"I can't imagine tomorrow. Don't be silly. We're going to live forever, and our kids will be best friends, too." We clinked our bottles of Old Style.

A few years later Patty was diagnosed with bone cancer. Other than dying, she worried most about losing her hair. I suppose she couldn't wrap her mind around half of her mandible disappearing much like—nearly thirty years later—I couldn't visualize losing a breast. But her hair, *that* she could imagine. In college, we spent countless hours styling our hair before track meets and parties. Rather, I spent hours styling her hair; mine was short and required less work, just mousse and a curling iron. She had an abundance of fine, wheat-blond hair. She used hot rollers faithfully; soft curls bounced on her shoulders.

I had moved to Houston a year before her diagnosis. Patty had had a couple of root canals that didn't dent the stabbing pain in her mouth, so her dentist sent her to a specialist for a biopsy. At the appointment, the oral surgeon told her it could be one of three things: an infection, some sort of bone disease, or cancer. Since we talked on the phone often and I had convinced myself her pain could be cleared up by strong antibiotics, I didn't suspect anything would be amiss when she called one night with the biopsy results. "Quigs, remember how I always said I would die young?"

"Yeah, remember how I always said you're full of shit?"

"I have cancer."

My mind raced for a different explanation, one that kept her alive. I stretched the phone cord into the bathroom and sank onto the toilet seat. "That doesn't mean you're going to die."

I flew from Houston to Chicago the weekend before her surgery to remove half of her mandible. We spent Friday and Saturday pretending everything was normal, as if I had come to celebrate an early Thanksgiving with my second family. Voices boomed as everyone talked over each other. She had seven siblings: seven big-boned German Southsiders and Patty, small and delicate compared to her brothers and sister. She had tiny hands and feet—size four-and-a-half compared to my size ten. Her strong jaw would set just so when she dug in to resist something, and her siblings would fall in line.

Because Patty's surgery would be so extensive, her doctor wanted to begin pre-op the night before surgery. Patty's fiancé, Vaughn, drove us to the hospital, and her mom sat in front beside him. I kept up a steady stream of chatter, trying to keep the mood light. Patty's laugh wavered in the car, but her mind drifted miles away. Christmas decorations hung from every streetlight and an odd red glow flamed against her face.

"My hair. The doctor said I'm going to lose my hair." She looked out her window.

I scrambled for something to say that wouldn't sound hollow or false. "Too bad I don't have that Halloween wig anymore. You'd look great as a Dallas Cowboy cheerleader."

"I don't have big boobs, though."

"Socks. I used firm rolled-up socks." I mock-grabbed my breasts as if they were 34DDs, instead of the 34As we both had. If she had lived, what would she have said to console me, take my mind off my surgeries? Probably something about my not needing a bra anymore or the possibility that I'd run faster without breasts getting in the way—not that mine did. If I had cried, she would have patted my back like she had in college when I was sobbing over a toilet, drunk and heartbroken about a break-up. "Don't cry. You're my rock. My Rock of Gibraltar."

Her mom had been listening. "We'll get you a wig, Patty. It'll look just like your real hair. Same color and everything."

We had driven by a wig store on 95th Street earlier that weekend. The huge window flaunted a battalion of mannequin heads bedecked with wigs of long, flowing hair in all different shades of blond, red, and brown, looking like a horde of decapitated prostitutes. Were conservative wigs for housewives, grandmothers, and cancer patients tucked in the back room, kind of like reverse pornography, the centerfolds on the outside? I nudged Patty. "Maybe we can get your wig on 95th. You can sample the latest hooker hairdos."

"Yeah right. I'll need some new clothes to perfect my look." Patty smiled at me.

Vaughn pulled up in front of the hospital to let us out. I picked up Patty's overnight bag and followed her and her mom inside. Patty's mom walked with her no-nonsense-let's-get-this-job-done attitude, much like she approached her job as a bookkeeper or being a mother to eight. Patty's surgery signified a puzzling entry on one of her spreadsheets, a problem to be solved and reconciled before moving on. The automatic doors whooshed behind us, signaling the end of Patty's days as a healthy runner, ushering her into a tenuous world of hope and despair. When we finally got to her room, Patty perched on the edge of her hospital bed, reluctant to claim the role of patient. Her mom sat on the chair near the window. That left me and Vaughn standing. I glanced at my watch—about an hour to kill before I had to leave for the airport.

"I can take you now, Quigs." Vaughn rattled the change in his pockets, trying to figure out what to do next. In motion, he didn't have to think about losing Patty.

"No. We still have time." I didn't want to leave Patty. I wanted to freeze time, maintaining the illusion of her whole and healthy. I wanted to lean back on the bed with her, eat popcorn, and watch one of her silly soap operas like we had in college. She had arranged her class schedule so she could follow Luke and Laura on *Guiding Light* before track practice.

"Do you want me to style your hair, Twink?" Her eyes lit up at my use of our nickname. One night in college we had worn the same outfit: denim overalls and white turtlenecks dotted with red hearts. One of the football guys working the food service line looked up and said, "What are you, a couple of Twinkies?" We chose it as our nickname and signed notes to each other "Twink" or "Twinkie." "I can do a few braids to keep your hair out of your face tomorrow. Whatever you want."

"How about a French braid down the middle?" She dug through her bag for her brush and comb. She held a ponytail holder in her hand as I ran my fingers through her hair, arranging it into three sections. I tried not to think about it falling out and wondered if I would ever style it again, but quickly swept that thought away. Her mom and Vaughn watched, lost in their own thoughts. I combed through each section to smooth the puckers, then balanced the comb on her right shoulder and quickly wove a braid along the top and back of her head, occasionally easing the comb through the sections. I wanted her hair to be perfect, one less thing to worry about.

My stomach churned, and I didn't want to leave. At dinner, Patty had picked at the food on her plate, absentmindedly pushing it around. Her stomach growled. She probably wanted to escape. Run fast and far away.

Vaughn stretched his arms as an excuse to check his watch. "We better go. Ma, do you want to stay here? I can come back."

I took a deep breath and squeezed Patty's shoulders. Everyone stood up. Patty had that expression she'd get before a track meet: lips pursed, quiet, intense, as if harnessing her energy. "You can all go. I'm tired. I need to sleep."

"I can stay, Patty," her mom said.

"No, it's ok, Ma, go home and try to sleep. I'll see you in the morning." Patty hugged her mom, then me. I stepped aside as Vaughn held her tight, burying his head in her hair, inhaling her. He sniffled. She stepped back and smiled, her eyes dancing as she wagged her finger at him. "Don't even think about it."

How many times had I heard her say that? "Don't even think about eating the last cookie.""Don't even think about..." whatever foolishness I was about to get us into. We were too young to say we loved each other, so I hugged her again. She would have teased me if I had said it. Best friends in the 80s didn't say they loved each other every day. We just did.

OCCASIONALLY, women dealing with cancer come to the spa where I work. They usually bring a gaggle of friends to celebrate the end of chemo. I admire the women who stand firm, their heads a shiny beacon of determination to confront cancer on their terms. I don't admire anyone less for wearing a wig or a turban, but I liked the idea of staring cancer in the face as if it were a duel—the medical team in one holster and a fuck-you-cancer attitude in the other. I used to think I would approach cancer the same way if I had to. Head-on. In your face. I wouldn't shy away from hair loss like Patty had. But she had been twenty-three. I was fifty-one.

MY NURSE SAID my hair would begin to fall out after the second round of chemo. As promised, a few days after my second infusion, dozens of short, silky strands fluttered onto my shoulders as I went about my day. Hundreds more slithered through my fingers and down the drain when I washed my hair. I didn't want to wake up one morning with clumps of hair on my pillow like a cicada's husk or the molt of a snake, no longer useful, but evoking the memory of my former self. I scheduled an appointment to have my head shaved and invited my mom and a couple of my friends to turn my appointment into a celebration. My stylist, Barb, had arranged to use the station overlooking the river, pivoting a couple of the reception chairs to face us, creating an island of support. I appreciated sitting at a different station; the specter of losing my hair wouldn't haunt every haircut to come.

While we waited for my mom, Maggie adjusted her camera, testing the lighting, training her camera on me, shifting her position to minimize backlighting from the bank of windows behind me. She had shot mother-son photos of me and Jake a few years earlier, and I trusted her tender, unflinching eye.

I glanced at my watch. "You can start, Barb. My mom's running late." I didn't add "per usual." She'd have an implausible, dramatic excuse: drawbridge raised, a telemarketer who wouldn't take no for an answer, or perhaps she fell asleep in the bathtub. She had a dysfunctional relationship with time. Long before cellphones were invented, my brothers and I used to tell her it was a good thing telephones didn't have cameras to record her lying. She conflated arrival time with departure time. Hair appointment at noon? Leave home at noon. Dinner reservations at six? Start the bathwater at six.

Barb adjusted the cape around my neck. Mom breezed into the salon, and I waved at her. She pecked me on the cheek. The acrid tang of smoke clung to her. She looked nervous, more nervous than I felt. Once I had decided to shave my head, I wanted to put it behind me, avoiding a long, drawn-out transition. As a child, I had wondered if swimming pool water would feel warmer if I gradually eased in one step at a time, allowing each inch of my body to acclimate. Or would the initial shock wear off quickly if I jumped in and began swimming? Eventually, I realized plunging in left me breathless for a moment, but the chill faded quickly. I hoped to blunt the impact of being bald by controlling my transformation. A dive rather than a step, when so much else was unpredictable.

Barb stood behind me as she had for all my haircuts. She rested her hands on my shoulders, and we looked in the mirror—my short, wavy hair—a grown-out version of the pixie cut we both loved. She combed her fingers through my hair gently, easing my tension. I wished she would say, "What are we going to do today?" like she had for ten years. Her eyes glimmered.

"Are you okay?" I asked. Her husband had died of cancer the previous year. I had selfishly not considered her possible pain.

She nodded and placed her left hand on top of my head, angling it down as she turned on the clipper and slid it up the back of my head. My fine hair offered little resistance. I felt like crying but didn't want to appear weak. I wasn't ready to look like someone who had cancer. Hell, I wasn't ready to have cancer, to be labeled a cancer patient. I thought I had come to terms with my tumor during my treatments and procedures to date, but the reality washed over me anew. I opened my eyes and looked at my lap. Brown and silver strands of hair shimmered against the black cape. I cupped my hands, catching some hair in my palms as it cascaded down the cape in small waves. Maggie circled us, shooting pictures from a variety of angles, pausing now and then to show my friends and Mom.

I looked up at the mirror, and my dad stared back at me. I sucked in a deep breath. I had always thought I resembled my mom more. My dad and I shared a strong, hawkish nose and angular jaw. Without hair to soften my angles, my face became interchangeable with his.

I glanced at my mom to see if she thought the same. I pointed to my head. "Hey, Mom, who do I look like?"

After the divorce, my brothers and I rarely saw our dad. He moved overseas and never thought to send us pictures. We missed a progression of photos showing him age. When we all finally reconnected at my grandmother's funeral, he was sixty-seven and had leapfrogged time, evolving from an ex-navy hippie to an old man in an instant. I had no idea what he had looked like in his early fifties. But, right then, staring at myself in the mirror, I knew how he would have looked if he'd stayed in the navy and how much of my identity fluttered to the floor as I transformed into a masculine version of myself.

If he were still alive, what would he have thought about my cancer? Would he have tried to be supportive? Or would he have taken refuge in the miles between us? As much as I would have wanted him to be the kind of dad who would hold my hand during chemo, I imagine he would have stayed somewhere with cheap rent and plenty of sunshine, sending little notes from time to time.

"You look just like your dad." My mom's chin quivered. I wanted to hug her, protect her, shield her from more loss. They had tried dating again after Grandma's funeral—ultimately the same two people who married each other in 1960—but more stubborn.

"Your dad must have been hot!" Jo laughed.

Barb hesitated before clipping the top of my head. I smiled in the mirror and nodded to reassure her. Perhaps I told myself it was okay to take this next step, that being bald and losing one more facet of femininity wouldn't matter to me. Barb ran the clipper across my scalp, and my hair tumbled onto the cape and around the chair. The salon hummed with the whir of blow dryers and chatter. If it had been quiet, maybe I could have heard my hair fall like snow on a still evening, a blanket of snow muting all other sound but descending snowflakes. Sometimes, it felt as if I participated in and witnessed my cancer simultaneously. Looking in the mirror magnified this split. I watched myself lose my hair while coming to terms with its loss.

Barb swished a soft brush over my scalp and face, tickling my nose and lips as fine hairs whispered onto the cape and ground. She swiveled the chair, checking for longer patches. I smiled at my friends and Mom.

"You look great!" Amy said and snapped some photos with her cellphone.

Jo rubbed my nubby scalp. "Sweetie, you have a beautiful head."

My mom rested her cheek against mine and wrapped her arms around me. I patted her shoulder, aware of Maggie leaning in for a closeup, conscious of a sudden hush in the salon. The stylists and customers seemed frozen in place. A few ladies swiped at tears, probably reliving their own cancer or that of someone they loved.

A knot wedged in my throat, and I looked down to avoid crying. I smoothed the purple fleece cap I'd been clutching like a stress ball. I stood up and hugged Barb. "Thank you."

She squeezed me tight. "No. Thank you."

I tugged on my cap and flashed two peace signs and a big smile at my personal paparazzi, eager to step out of the limelight. From force of habit, I slid my fingers under my cap to straighten my hair. Fine razor stubble tugged at the fleece. No more hat head for a while.

"Who wants coffee? Paradigm anyone?" I felt giddy, relieved, another item to cross off my cancer checklist.

"My treat!" my mom said. She zipped her coat and fumbled in her purse for cigarettes.

Of all the coffeehouses in Sheboygan, Paradigm was a safe place to experiment with being bald. It is a refuge for angsty teenagers, stay-at-home moms, businesspeople, artists, and small-town bohemians who like good music, fresh gluten-free pastries, and strong coffee. After we ordered our coffee and treats, I removed my cap and smoothed my fingers over my head. It felt downy as I stroked toward my neck, but when I rubbed toward the top of my head, the bristles tugged as if going against the grain of freshly sanded wood. Amy took more pictures to post on Facebook. I looked at the images, absorbing what my friends and mom were coming to terms with, knowing I could pull them up later and imprint them on my mind. Me bald. Smiling. Tucking fear away. I felt jittery and couldn't tell if my anti-nausea meds or the rollercoaster emotions of being shorn caused my jangly nerves. Probably both.

I'M SURE I wasn't the only one who barely slept the night before Patty's operation. I imagined a collective anxious vigil—her mom fingering her rosary in bed, Vaughn pacing, and me more than a thousand miles away, staring at my ceiling, ineffective. The surgeon removed Patty's left mandible and wired her jaw shut. On days when she was lucid and not in too much pain, she held the phone to her ear as I babbled about work, some guy I had a crush on, or anything that required little input from her. We worked out a system where she tapped on the phone once for no, twice for yes, and three times if she wanted to laugh.

"Do you need anything?"

Tap.

"Do you need to rest?"

Tap. Tap.

"Are you in pain?"

Tap.

"Would you lie to me?"

Tap. Tap.

"I knew it. I always knew you were a big, fat liar."

Tap. Tap. Tap.

"Would it be easier for you if I mail little notes until you can talk again?"

Tap. Tap.

"Okay. I'll do that. Do you want me to come visit?"

Tap. Tap.

Instead, Patty and Vaughn came to visit me in April. Five months of my life running ahead while hers stalled. Five months of pretending everything would go back to normal. I had gotten involved with a local theatre group, and we were staging *Death Takes a Holiday*. It had devolved into a campy melodrama, much to the director's dismay.

After dress rehearsal, I sped to the airport. I had wanted to meet Patty and Vaughn at the gate but instead met them on their way to baggage claim. If not for Vaughn, I would have run past them without recognizing Patty. I hadn't realized how much her jaw had defined her. Her wig swallowed her face. She cocked her head to the left like a little bird tucking its beak into its wing. Her left cheek puffed out like a squirrel's nut-filled jowl, and the area where her jawbone should have been collapsed inward.

"Twink! Vaughn!" I hugged Patty tight, careful to put my head next to the right side of her face. Her wig tickled my nose and smelled like her shampoo. That surprised me. My mom had worn falls and frosted wigs when they were all the rage in the early 70s. They always smelled like cigarette smoke and cologne, vaguely plastic. My brothers and I used to try them on, pretending to audition for the *Carol Burnett Show*.

"You look great!" I said with as much sincerity as I could muster.

"You're such a liar." Her voice wobbled as her tongue navigated the space left by her missing teeth. How did I not realize she would lose teeth along with her mandible?

"It's great to see you." Vaughn hugged me. Patty's cancer had made us allies. When they began dating, she stopped going to parties, and I resented the time they spent together even though I had a boyfriend, too. Vaughn proposed after I moved to Texas. Patty's diagnosis stalled their wedding plans. No looking at wedding gowns. No picking out bridesmaids' dresses. No choosing anything pretty.

"Let's get your bags and go home. Hungry? Tired? Thirsty?"

"Slooooow down," Patty laughed. "We're fine. We ate on the plane."

We drove with the windows open, and they marveled at the balmy air. Winter liked to linger in Chicago, but Houston had shrugged it off in February like an ill-fitting coat.

The next day we went to NASA and Galveston. Patty had always liked sunbathing and would get a warm coppery glow. Chemo had made her skin thin and beige. The skies glowered, and the wind pelted us with millions of grains of sand while we tried to relax on the deserted beach. Bathing suits were not an option. I doubted Patty had brought one; it would have fallen off. She probably needed to shop in the girls' department.

Vaughn looked up and down the beach. "Where is everyone?"

"Texans think this weather is too cold."

"It *is* a little windy," Patty zipped her windbreaker. The little pink scar from her tracheotomy peeked above her jacket, and I cursed cancer for chipping away at so much of her.

"Are you cold?"

"A little bit. I have to go to the bathroom."

I pointed at a large bathhouse. "Is that too far?"

She shook her head and fiddled with her wig. She rested her hand near her ear—ready to catch the wig if a gust caught it. We shook the sand from our beach towels as we walked to the bathhouse. Vaughn held the towels while Patty and I went inside. A line of stalls stood open. After peeing, we flushed, then washed our hands at the row of sinks, a shiny metal fake mirror above them. I smiled and waved a peace sign at our murky reflections. We almost looked normal. Patty stuck out her tongue at me and adjusted her wig in the mirror.

"Frick. It's filled with sand."

"Just take it off and shake it out."

Her eyebrows flew up as if I had suggested she run naked into the surf.

"It's okay. I don't think anyone's in here."

Patty took off the wig and shook it like a stuffed animal. Grains of sand pinged the floor until a small mound of sand had piled near her feet. Her hair had begun to grow in and was almost a half-inch long—soft and light brown.

"Jeez! Did you leave some sand on the beach?"

She giggled and gave her wig another shake. A lady exited one of the stalls, and her gaze ricocheted from Patty's nearly bald head to the wig in her hands and back to Patty's head. The lady's mouth gaped open, her jaw flapping up and down like a guppy's. She left without washing her hands. Patty and I burst out laughing.

"You don't need that wig, Twink. Your hair is adorable."

"Really?"

"Really. You look like Mia Farrow. I'll cut mine that short after the play."

She stuffed the wig in my tote bag, and we walked out of the bathhouse still giggling about the lady's reaction. Vaughn turned around as he heard us laughing. "Well, well, well." He beamed at Patty. It felt like we had all jumped a hurdle together, one step closer to healing.

At the time, I had no idea how hard each milestone was for her or anyone with cancer. I had no concept of the daily struggle to reclaim one's body, one's identity. It had been more difficult for Patty because it impacted her face. Her prosthesis blistered her gums, so she rarely wore it. Years later, with my own cancer, I wore loose-fitting, wildly patterned shirts to camouflage my missing breast, rarely wearing the mastectomy bras with my silicone breast form. I could wear a bra or go without and—depending on what I wore—nobody would know. In college, there were few secrets or off-limit topics, but after her diagnosis, I never asked if she and Vaughn made love after her surgery, if they kissed after she had somewhat healed, or how she felt about her femininity—nothing. I only said "when you get better"—that far-off when—without defining better.

I FELT NERVOUS about Jake's reaction to my baldness. After my diagnosis, I began a blog to avoid repeating an endless litany of treatments and side effects when friends and family called to check on me; and, more importantly, my blog posts sheltered Jake from the daily reality of cancer. Hair loss would be hard to hide, unless I wore a wig, which I didn't want to do. They never looked real, no matter how hard the stylists tried to make the wig similar to the patient's last hairstyle.

Thanks to Facebook, Jake saw the photos Amy had posted. He hadn't wanted to go to the salon, begging off for school and work. Perhaps seeing the photos first desensitized him, allowing him to come to terms with my baldness at his own pace. After the initial shock of my diagnosis, he kept his feelings to himself. As it turned out, my lack of hair didn't faze him. When he got home from work, he rubbed my scalp and said, "Sweet!" The next night, Jake and his friend, Nate, shaved their heads. When he came home, we stood in our kitchen and took a selfie, huge smiles, middle fingers up, flipping off cancer.

A parade of polar vortices pummeled the upper Midwest that winter. I wore knit or polar fleece beanies constantly—sometimes two at a time—even to bed. My nurse gave me a prescription for a "cranial prosthesis," as if I could go to a pharmacy to buy a fake head. I keep the prescription as a memento or maybe as insurance against recurrence. It has expired, so it's as useless as a wig would have been at disguising chemotherapy's effect on me.

Every night, after tucking Jake in, I consulted the internet for information about new symptoms I experienced and how to mitigate them. Unsurprisingly, there were many camps on the message boards about hair loss: the wig at all costs—usually for younger or married women; the half-hearted wig contingent—women who only wore their wigs outside the home; and no wigs ever—women like me. A few women said they had used cold caps to prevent or minimize hair loss. Cold caps hadn't been covered in any of the information my nurses had provided.

Chemo destroys rapidly dividing cells, such as cancer. Unfortunately, skin, hair, and nails also divide quickly and become collateral damage in chemo's quest to eliminate or stall cancer. The nurses urged me to chew on ice chips to constrict blood vessels in my mouth, thereby decreasing mouth sores. Although I chomped on them constantly on chemo Mondays, my mouth molted. No sores. Just peeling skin as if the inside of my cheeks had been sunburned. Cold caps are snug, chilled caps to wear during chemo treatments that work much the same way ice chips do. With the ice chips, the cool stream of intravenous drugs and flushes, and the polar vortices, I couldn't tolerate the prospect of one more thing that would chill me to the bone. I didn't see anyone use cold caps at the cancer center, and the nurses I asked said they didn't think they were that effective. In 2015—the year after I went through chemo—the FDA approved the use of cold caps, but insurance companies still don't cover the expense. Since men can go bald with impunity, cold caps are probably considered a frivolous expense.

Even the cancer support boards bring out the trolls. Some women disparaged the use of cold caps and posted comments like, "It's just hair. It'll grow back," when women asked about them. Other women stepped in to remind the know-it-alls that each woman has her own journey, her own choices. Frigging journey. Frigging support groups. Even though I knew my hair would grow back, I remembered how devastating hair loss had been for Patty. I hope I hadn't minimized her suffering by telling her it would grow back. Knowing something intellectually is not the same as knowing it viscerally.

BY MAY, Patty's cancer metastasized to her pelvic bones, and she needed radiation again. In June, I flew to Chicago to spend a few days with her. On the way to her radiation appointment, she pulled up to a stoplight, and a man in a semitruck to our right whistled and said, "Helloooo ladies."

I waved at him through my open window.

Patty said, "He only whistled because he couldn't see my face." She didn't sound bitter, just wistful.

"He was checking out your legs. If he had seen your face, he would have fallen in love with you."

Until I had my own cancer, my own transformation, I didn't understand how much the little slights accumulated and hurt, chiseling away at my confidence.

She knew the hospital as if it were her favorite shopping mall. She smiled and waved at people she recognized, leaving a chorus of "Hi Patty" in our wake. The radiation waiting room felt like a dungeon or a fortress, the thick cement-block walls shielding us from harm. A technician opened a door and called Patty's name. She stood up and wagged her finger at me. "Don't even think about picking up a doctor."

"Now you're talking." I winked at her. Before the door closed, I heard her ask about the technician's kids. Classic Patty—shy, but warm, always putting people at ease. I pulled a book out of my purse and pretended to read. I gave up and rested my head in my hands and offered up some sort of prayer, more of a lament. Why Patty? Why not an asshole? The door to the waiting room opened, and a lady wheeled a stroller into the waiting room. She lifted a toddler—probably her daughter—out of the stroller and held the little girl on her lap. The girl nestled against the woman's chest. Fresh graffiti-like scars were scribbled on the girl's bare scalp. The mother tucked her chin around the girl's head like a mother bird wrapping her wing around her fledglings, keeping them warm and safe. She inhaled. I nodded at her, and her lips twisted into something like a smile, terrible and wry. I looked at my book, and the words swam in front of my eyes. Why that little girl? Why Patty? Why?

The door sighed open, releasing Patty into the room, into a bit more of life. I stood up and stuffed my book into my purse. "Does it hurt?"

She shook her head. "I'm getting tan down there."

"You rebel. I bet you've been lying out naked."

We drove back to her house; it was hot and muggy outside, and the air-conditioner in the kitchen barely cooled the air. Heat sucked every ounce of energy from her, so we curled up on the basement couch to watch a movie. Patty clicked on the remote and found one of the movie channels. *Terms of Endearment* was about to start. I told her she'd love it. I had been watching it every couple of weeks since Patty's diagnosis, using it as an excuse to cry. Patty tapped her long fingernails against the remote, and I cringed. I grabbed the remote and turned off the movie. I have no idea why I thought she would love a movie about a young woman dying from cancer, even if it wasn't bone cancer.

"Crap, Patty, I'm sorry. That was stupid. We should watch a soap opera."

"Yeah right. Or a baseball game. At least we don't know how they'll turn out."

"It's just a movie. You're going to live."

"If I do, I won't be able to have kids. The radiologist told me my ovaries are getting too much radiation." How long had she known and not said anything?

"Can't they cover them with something like the dentist does?"

"They're too close to my pelvic bones. Will you have a baby for me if I live?"

"If you live? Of course, you're going to live."

She looked at me, challenging me to lie to her face or look away. "If I live, will you?" Desperation crept into her voice.

"Of course. Does this mean I get to sleep with Vaughn?"

"Don't even think about it." She flicked me with her fingernails. "Turkey baster for you."

I hated that she thought about living as a possibility instead of a reality. We all talked about a future with her in it. I would say, "When you're done with this shit, we'll go to Paris." Vaughn would tell her, "When you're finished with your treatments, we'll get married." Her sister, Rosie, mentioned flea market adventures. Patty would nod but didn't buy any bridal magazines or hang the poster of the Eiffel Tower I'd sent her. She had been mentally preparing for a premature death for a long time. As much as I wanted to believe she would survive, I knew she wouldn't. I didn't know much about cancer then, but the little I understood about hers didn't leave much hope. By the time of my diagnosis, the internet had demystified cancer statistics. My odds were much greater than Patty's had ever been.

In August, I flew to Chicago for a weekend visit with Patty. Her fatigue didn't leave much space for anything other than resting. I can't remember if she was in treatment at the time, or if her doctors were stalling, not quite holding out false hope, but not stating a prognosis. Maybe they had told her, and she kept it to herself, like a dark secret gnawing at her. In the two months since my last visit, she had aged twenty years. Her sallow skin stretched taut across her cheekbones. Vaughn had bought her a puppy as if to coax her into staying alive—if not for him and the rest of us—then at least for the puppy. The puppy nipped at everyone's feet and tumbled around the kitchen wrestling with Millie, their old German Shepherd. Millie hid under the kitchen table, unimpressed.

Vaughn looked at me. "Can you believe Patty has never been to a Cubs game?"

"This is the South Side." Chicago baseball allegiance aligned geographically with an invisible and occasionally shifting line on the map determining which team people followed.

One of Patty's brothers snorted. "Our old man would roll over in his grave if he heard you were gonna take Patty to a Cubs game."

"Wanna go?" Vaughn asked. His determination to find new experiences for her made me see him through her eyes. Sweet, steady, kind.

"Sure. If Patty's game, I'm cool with it."

"I've always wanted to see Wrigley Field," she said.

The term 'bucket list' hadn't been coined in 1986. If it had, I wouldn't have guessed a Cubs game scored high on Patty's list. I suppose as she became more aware of her mortality and her cancer continued to expand, distances contracted. Paris was no longer an option. Wrigley Field would have to do.

"Can we get tickets?" I asked.

"We'll scalp them." Vaughn rested his palms on Patty's shoulders and kissed the top of her head, resting his cheek against her soft curls. Tears prickled my nose; I picked up the puppy and smothered her with kisses until she wiggled out of my arms.

My flight was scheduled for late evening, so we went to the Sunday afternoon game. Night games didn't begin until 1988, a source of pride or contention depending on who you talked to. Saturday tickets were usually harder to scalp—the games an excuse for a raucous pre-party to the drunken scene in Wrigleyville. Sundays had a more relaxed, family-friendly vibe.

It was a perfect summer day in Chicago. The sun glimmered on the lake, and a cool breeze blew from the east. I had borrowed one of Patty's sweatshirts. Summer in Houston is a steamy sauna, and my blood must have thinned. Goosebumps dappled my arms and legs while we waited for Vaughn to buy tickets from a man shepherding a flock of developmentally delayed adults. We wound our way up ramp after ramp, pausing at each level so Patty could rest, until I thought we couldn't go any higher.

"Next stop, Heaven," I said and then mentally kicked myself. Would I ever learn to keep my mouth shut?

"At least two of my favorite people will be with me." Patty smiled, rescuing me.

When we finally reached our seats, Vaughn arranged the pillow Patty had brought from home to cushion her butt. She had lost so much muscle mass that her bones ached when she sat on hard seats. During the seventh inning stretch, Vaughn took a picture of us. Our heads rested against each other with my arm draped around her shoulders. She felt as fragile as a hummingbird. The bones in her knees stood in sharp relief against my muscular thighs. Her cheek caved in where her prosthesis should have been—where her jawbone should have been. She smiled at the camera, gentle and knowing, her lips closed, without her fresh-faced, straight-toothed grin from college. My expression? Bittersweet yet happy, happy to have one more afternoon with her. Yet impending loss softens my eyes. That day, at Wrigley Field, Vaughn and I pretended Patty would live. We talked about the following summer and the summer after that; we told her we could go wherever she wanted.

TWINKIES

She smiled but didn't say anything about the future beyond my upcoming visit after Labor Day.

When they dropped me off at O'Hare, I hugged Patty and wouldn't let her go. "I love you, Twink. I'm going to miss you." I buried my face in her shoulder.

"I'm not going anywhere."

"I know. I meant these next few weeks."

But I knew. I knew she probably wouldn't be alive when I returned. When I hugged Vaughn, I whispered, "Keep me posted." I waved as they drove off, watching his car fade around the curve. After I left, Patty spiraled, and her muscles wasted away. She could no longer manage the stairs to her bedroom and slept with her mom in the master bedroom off the kitchen. I called her every night after I got home from work.

"My mom is dousing me with holy water in the middle of the night."

"That's hilarious." Her mom had dragged her to a faith healer at a church somewhere in Chicago. She would have sacrificed chickens, baby lambs, anything to keep Patty alive.

"Someone brought it back from Medjugorje."

"It's probably from the Chicago River."

Her mom squawked in the background, "Don't make fun of that water. It's holy water."

"Okay, okay, Ma. I'm sure it's gonna work."

By the end of August, Patty no longer came to the phone. She never complained, but from what I've read, bone cancer is painful. The last time I saw her, she asked me to massage her scalp. Everyone else was afraid to hurt her. Her skull felt like a sack of marbles. She told me not to worry, that one of her cousins had cysts on her head, too. I didn't think they were cysts; they didn't move. Vaughn told me her last scan showed tumors riddling her bones.

The day before my scheduled flight in September, Vaughn called me at work, "Hey, Quigs, she's gone."

I sucked in my breath and clutched the phone.

"Are you okay?"

I nodded my head as if he could see me. I squeaked out a yes and exhaled. "I'll change my flight and call you with the info."

My nose had filled with snot, and I sniffled it in. I set my head on my desk, pressing my forehead into the cool wood. I heard footsteps and lifted my head as Red, the president of the company, walked past my desk. I tried to brush away my tears.

"What's wrong with you? You look like your best friend just died."

"She did."

His normally florid face flushed even deeper red. Nicknames in the south are short and accurate. I pushed my chair back and ran to the bathroom. He must have tracked down my friend, Beth, to check on me. She found me in the bathroom and stood behind me, patting me on the back while I doused my face with cold water.

"Patty?"

"Mm hmm."

"I'm so sorry. At least she's not suffering anymore."

"I know. I'm just going to miss her."

"Why don't you go home? Maybe you can get an earlier flight."

A box of chocolates and a note lay on my typewriter. Red must have immediately taken the elevator to the lobby to buy a peace offering. I knocked on my boss's door. Her light blue eyes—usually flinty—softened when she saw me. She must have heard the entire exchange. "Red's an ass. I'm sorry about your friend. You go on home and get yourself to Chicago."

SOME STUBBORN HAIRS remained in my scalp and snagged in my beanies like leg hairs poking through tights. I envied Sinead O'Connor's shiny bald look. Maybe her photos had been airbrushed. The razor stubble drove me bonkers. Jake hated wearing dog hair—unavoidable with two shedding dogs—so he had lint rollers in the bathroom, his bedroom, and car. Our house has only one small bathroom, crammed with a clawfoot bathtub, pedestal sink, toilet, and cabinet. It wasn't uncommon for all four of us to be in the bathroom at the same time—the dogs, me, and Jake. One day while Jake was getting ready for school, I sat on top of the toilet seat chatting with him. He ran the lint roller over his polar fleece and barked at Sophie to stay away from him. When Jake removed the outer roll of masking tape on the lint roller, Sophie's two-inch-long blond hairs and Rowdy's short, spiky black hairs blanketed the tape.

"Hey, I have an idea. Let me use that." I held out my hand.

Jake looked curious. He knew I didn't care about the dog hair, that I viewed it as a tradeoff for the dogs' unconditional love. I stood next to him facing the mirror and was struck afresh by how much we looked alike. With our fuzzy heads, the resemblance had grown stronger. I ran the lint roller over my head in all directions. I held it out for inspection; the tape was flecked with hundreds of little hairs randomly scattered like hieroglyphs or animal tracks.

From that point on, I rolled my scalp every day until hair no longer peppered the tape. Judging from the patches of stubble in no obvious pattern, the chemo would not have made me completely bald.

Spring eased into Sheboygan, and I finally went without a cap on warm days. People glanced at me, then slid their eyes to something, someone safe. The gray middle ground of polite indifference did not exist. I felt invisible most of the time. One day, while I waited in line at Walgreen's, I observed the cashier making inane conversation with each customer in the long line ahead of me. The girl shouted over three customers' heads, "Did you shave your head because you wanted to, or are you making some kind of statement?"

The people in front of me swiveled to gauge my reaction. An awkward silence bloomed around us, and I realized she must have been speaking to me. I was so accustomed to being looked through,

I assumed she had asked someone else. Nobody ahead of me was bald. She looked directly at me and repeated her question.

"I have cancer," I said.

"Oh, well, you know, some people just like to shave their heads."

"Oh, well, you know, some people just have cancer."

She continued ringing up the people in front of me while prattling away. "Oh. Cancer. Do you lose your hair when you have cancer?" Did she ever think before opening her mouth?

I felt like her personal cancer infomercial. I remained patient. "Sometimes. It depends on what kind of chemotherapy you receive."

I hoped she would be more sensitive in the future, but I doubted it. What did the other people in line think? Did they mind being ignored while she rang their purchases? Were they amused? Angry? Pitying? I wondered what my mom would have done if she had been with me. Probably track down the manager.

"Well, if I ever have cancer, I'll make 'em give me stuff that lets me keep my hair."

"That's a good idea." I nodded as if she had said something profound.

I sat in my car and shook my head. Did that happen to other cancer patients? Fear of interactions like that probably drove some women to wear wigs. With a wig, they could trick themselves and others into thinking everything was normal.

A JUMBLE of drunken relatives and friends had crammed into Patty's home by the time I arrived. My grandfather used to quip that the only difference between an Irish wedding and an Irish wake was one less mouth to feed. It seemed true for Germans as well. Everyone was telling and retelling Patty stories, easing their pain with humor.

I slept in Patty's bed that weekend. Her sheets smelled of the same detergent she used in college. If I inhaled deeply, vestiges of her favorite cologne, buried deep within her pillow, left a spicy

Opium-scented ghost behind. Patty's sister, Rosie, slept in the twin bed across the room. I stared at the ceiling, listening to Rosie breathe, feeling the loss of Patty beside me. We used to cram into her twin bed after parties. My roommate was a jock who was sound asleep before ten. I didn't feel like I belonged in my room. Patty's roommate didn't mind if we woke her up as long as we passed out quickly.

The following morning, Patty's mom gave each of us a list of things to do. She asked me to write the petitions for the Mass. She wanted me to read them; I had no idea how I would get through them.

Before the wake opened to the public, the funeral director arranged a private showing for the family. Patty's mom grabbed my elbow and insisted I was family. We all walked into the room—Patty's mom, brothers and sister, their wives and boyfriend, Vaughn, me, and her favorite aunt and uncle. I couldn't avoid looking at Patty. I needed to convince myself that she was irretrievably gone.

"No. It's wrong. All wrong. That doesn't look like Patty." Her mom shook her head, clearly agitated.

The funeral director stepped quietly toward her. Patty's mom insisted he remove the prosthesis because it made Patty's mouth look funny. We left the room while he made the adjustment. When we returned, I could see Patty's mom had been right. Patty had rarely worn the prosthesis, so it distorted her face, turning her into a stranger. She squeezed my arm again. "Her makeup's all wrong. Did you bring your makeup?"

I nodded my head. She had asked me to bring it just in case. It was a "just in case" I couldn't imagine so I'd agreed. When I was in grade school, I'd taught myself how to print left-handed just in case I lost my right arm. I understood "just in case," but I didn't think I would need to use my makeup. I approached Patty's casket and took my cosmetic bag out of my purse. It contained the same makeup we had worn in college; we didn't know we were supposed to throw makeup away after a year. I swabbed the iridescent blue, pink, and lavender shadows on her lids. I swooshed shimmery pink blush on her cheekbones. Patty's mom stood beside me, as if supervising. In my head, I heard the Donna Summers album we danced to while getting ready for parties. I put the blush away and took a deep breath.

"Go on. You're doing a great job," her mom encouraged me. The room behind us grew quiet as everyone watched. I wanted a beer. I wanted Patty to laugh with me about how serious everyone was. I could hear her jest, "You'd think I had died or something!"

I rested my pinky finger on her cheekbone and traced the blue eyeliner above her eyelashes. I am not religious, but I prayed her eyelids wouldn't flip open. They barely moved. Had they been glued or sewn shut? Not knowing simultaneously comforted and disturbed me. Her skin felt cool and immobile, and I felt as if I were painting a papier-mâché mask.

"Don't forget lipstick." Her mom leaned over the casket to inspect my handiwork.

I dabbed Patty's favorite pink gloss over the lipstick the mortician had chosen, trying not to tug against her mouth. I knew I couldn't hurt her, but her mouth had been through so much. I didn't want to inflict any posthumous pain.

"Yes, now she looks like herself." Patty's mom clutched my arm.

I exhaled, not realizing I had been holding my breath. I leaned in and whispered, "You owe me big time, Twink. Big time." I stepped back and looked at her, shrunken and doll-like on the satin padding. I didn't want to know how much weight she had lost. We had worn the same size in college. Her short wavy hair made her look like Joan of Arc. The mortician had strung Patty's confirmation rosary through her hands. The beads—artfully looped, the cross aligned with her chin—seemed staged, an impersonation of death.

Vaughn looked unmoored. We all did after so much time hoping, praying, and not thinking about the future. The future meant Patty was gone.

DURING MY TREATMENT, I often thought about Patty and her brief battle with cancer. The odds were stacked against her the entire time. Her type of bone cancer normally afflicts young men in their long bones such as their femurs. Amputation and aggressive chemotherapy and radiation can help treat cancer in the extremities, but it's hard to amputate a head and have a high survival rate. By the time I was diagnosed in 2013, so many advances had been made in treating all cancers, particularly breast cancer. Breast cancer is one hundred times more common than Patty's type of bone cancer, and, of course, the survival rate is much higher.

Patty never lost her eyebrows and eyelashes. My eyebrows and lashes fell out while I received Taxol, making me look like more of a cancer patient or a Conehead.

Rosie invited me and Jake to her house for Easter. It had been a long time—too long—since I had seen Patty's family, maybe five or six years. Maybe more. Jake had been a week old the last time they saw him and the seventeen-year leap from infant to teenager amazed them. They folded us into their Easter celebration as if no time had passed, catching us up on all the family news. Everyone treated Jake as if he were a long-lost grandson or nephew. Rosie and her husband, Larry, are avid Green Bay Packers fans—an oddity in Chicagoland—and had converted their spare bedroom into a Packers shrine. Larry proudly showed Jake his memorabilia. Patty's mom had a large box wrapped for me and insisted I sit in the living room to open it. I knew whatever was in the box would turn me into a puddle. I took the lid off and removed Patty's college track jacket. I had donated mine years earlier to a homeless shelter. Tears floated in my eyes. "There's more," her mom said.

I slid a black leather pouch from under the jacket. I opened it and looked up, surprised.

Her mom nodded. "Patty's pearls. She planned to wear them at her wedding."

"Are you sure? What about one of her nieces? Jacki?"

She shook her head, "Patty would have wanted you to have them."

"I suppose I'll have to get married."

"It's probably too late," Rosie said.

We all laughed. We drove away, Jake and I waving at Rosie and Patty's mom as they stood on the front porch, leaning into each other. Jake nudged my thigh. "I'm glad we came. I can see why you wanted me to meet them."

"Yeah, they've always treated me like family."

Jake rested his head against the window and fell asleep, leaving me with my memories. Had my baldness reminded them of Patty? Maybe enough years had passed, allowing their grief to fade to a dull ache, as mine had. My mind wandered to when we met in 1980, and I flipped through a six-year mental photo album of memories: racing at track meets; stealing the donut delivery from the dining hall; learning how to dance at parties with the basketball guys; skipping classes to shop in Chicago; running up the ski hill with our coach yelling "lean, dammit, lean"; drinking too much at parties and rescuing each other from unwanted advances; renting our first apartment together; styling her hair; scrawling the word 'Twinkies' in fresh cement on the way home from a party; saying goodbye at the airport the month before she died.

When my mind strayed to the image of her emaciated and weakened, I flipped past that memory. She would have wanted me to remember her laughing and running. She had visited my dreams for years, pointing her finger and admonishing me, "Don't even think about it." For years, it meant don't date men who turned out to be losers. Then, after my diagnosis, she snuck into my dreams and cautioned me against wondering if I, too, would die.

I HAD NEVER been fast—not like Patty—nicknamed White Lightning by a girl she raced in high school. I always had a pair of running shoes—nothing serious—until I trained for my first half marathon a couple of years before my diagnosis. The race organizers gave each runner two bibs—one for the front with our name on it and one for our backs that said, "I run for…" I wrote "Twinkies." Running became my lodestar throughout chemo—another marathon my goal. I ran two, then burnt out. After the Chicago Marathon, I felt defeated by my slow pace. Days passed. My running shoes gathered dog hair by the front door as autumn dwindled. I knew my desire would vanish altogether if I didn't run before snow fell. I had many conversations with myself as I walked my dogs, invariably bitching myself out about how grateful I should be to be alive, that I *could* run, that shaving thirty minutes off my time to qualify for Boston again was possible.

On a crisp November day, the sun gleamed low in the sky. I put on my running clothes and laced up my shoes: one for Patty, one for me. Rowdy followed me to the door, eager for a walk. I nuzzled his snout, then pulled on my windbreaker and mittens. I chided myself for waiting so long, my legs and lungs protesting. It had only been a month since the race, and my conditioning had evaporated. One foot in front of the other, breath by breath, I found my rhythm. The familiar three-mile loop didn't require thought, leaving my mind free to wonder. Would Patty have run marathons with me? Or would marathons have been my thing and short bursts of speed hers?

FOR YEARS, I took an aromatase inhibitor to prevent estrogen from being produced by my muscles and fat. After menopause—natural or, in my case, surgical—muscles and fat take over estrogen production. Estrogen, for the most part, is beneficial. Without it, women are prone to osteoporosis, dementia, cardiac issues, vaginal atrophy, as well as a whole host of other issues. I blame any new physical ailment on my medication. Before beginning the medicine, my oncologist ordered a baseline bone density scan. Each year, my numbers declined. He suggested I begin taking a bisphosphonate to stimulate bone growth. Otherwise, I'm at risk for fracture in my lumbar spine, femurs, and pelvis. He mentioned, almost offhand, that a rare side effect is osteonecrosis of the jaw. I didn't need him to define it. Osteo: bone. Necrosis: death.

"No."

"The risk is small." He seemed surprised by my quick retort.

"I know what someone looks like without a jawbone. My best friend had bone cancer in her left mandible. She died."

"But this isn't cancer."

"I know. But I only have one jaw." I felt entitled to a bit of unreasonable logic.

At each follow-up appointment, Dr. Lam encouraged me to continue taking the aromatase inhibitor beyond the five years we had initially discussed and to reconsider the bisphosphonate. I have always counted down for special events or steps in a challenge: how many bedtimes until Christmas; how many miles left in each race I've run; and now, how many years left of taking a medication that is eating holes in my bones.

I wondered what Patty would have done. She lost her mandible before the rest of her bones were consumed by cancer. The aromatase inhibitor I take has honeycombed my lumbar bones with each passing year. The bisphosphonate could simultaneously increase my bone density while also destroying my mandible. Now, before I drift into dreams, I ask Patty to help me decide what to do. I half expect her to appear, perching on the edge of my bed, wagging her finger at me, and saying, "Don't even think about it" before she vanishes, leaving me with an unanswered question, an unclear path to run alone.

Acknowledgements

In June 2015, I tossed a stone into a kettle at the Interlochen Writers Retreat. I am grateful for: Anne-Marie Oomen's pinch of prose; Katey Schultz's tutelage in chopping, slicing, and egging me on to dig deeper in my recipe files; Patricia Ann McNair's prodding and coaxing me to concoct complex yet simple stews; Chris Rice's belief that my dark and disparate ingredients belonged in Hypertext Magazine; instructors at Columbia College, Chicago and Interlochen for spicy craft talks; Kate Lebo's and Kase Johnstun's virtual prose-cooking shows; Michelle Latiolais and Raymond Obstfeld, my first writing teachers, for turning on the flame under the kettle years ago; my writing friends Nancy Parshall, Julia Poole, Gail Wallace Bozzano, Jen Gravley, Doro Boehme, and many more for the garlic and umami that inspire me; Joanne Grabinski's endowed scholarship—the icing on my cake; Dawn Newton's editorial skills, standing by the stove with me to heighten the flavor (with a healthy helping of commas); and countless friends and family who have eaten at my table and survived. I have boundless gratitude for residencies at Ragdale Foundation and Chef Linda's culinary creations which fueled my late-night writing sessions, and for Michigan Writers Cooperative Press. A million thanks for the enduring gift of Patty's friendship and letting me share her family, my mom's love and encouragement, and for Jake—the best bun in the oven, ever.

About the Judge

Michigan Writers Cooperative Press would like to express our thanks to DAWN NEWTON. Dawn is the author of *The Remnants of Summer*, a novel, and *Winded: A Memoir in Four Stages*, which details her ongoing dance with stage IV lung cancer. She was trained as a fiction writer and received scholarships to attend Michigan State University and Johns Hopkins University. Dawn has taught literature, creative writing, and composition at several colleges and in K-12 classrooms in Virginia and Michigan. She has three grown children—Rachel, Connor, and Nathaniel—and lives with her husband, Tim Dalton, and their dog, Clover, in East Lansing, Michigan.

About the Author

Kathleen Quigley is a writer and massage therapist living in Wisconsin yet dreaming of retiring someplace warm. She has been published in *Hypertext Review, Stoneboat Literary Journal, The Seventh Wave,* and *HerStry.blg,* among others. After pursuing an MFA in Creative Writing at Columbia College Chicago, Kathleen took a hiatus to raise her son and run marathons. She has been awarded residencies at Ragdale Foundation and is completing a memoir which explores mortality, femininity, and reclaiming identity after illness. Humor—sometimes screwball, often dark—infuses her writing. She loves all things purple and her crazy rescue dog.

About Michigan Writers Cooperative Press

This book was published in the spring of 2023 in a signed edition of 100 copies.

This chapbook is part of the Cooperative Series of the Michigan Writers Small Press Project, which was launched in 2005 to give members of Michigan Writers, Inc. a new avenue to publication. All of the chapbooks in this series are an author's first book in that genre. The Cooperative Press shoulders the publishing costs for the first edition, and writers share the marketing and promotional responsibilities in return for the prestige of being published by a press that prints only carefully selected manuscripts.

Chapbook length manuscripts of poetry, short stories, and essays are solicited each year from members and adjudicated by a panel of experienced writers and a judge who is a specialist in a particular genre. For more information, please visit www.michwriters.org.

MICHIGAN WRITERS is an open-membership organization dedicated to providing opportunities for networking, professional growth, and publication for writers of all ages and skill levels in Northwest Michigan and beyond.

MANAGING EDITOR: Gail Wallace Bozzano

BOOK DESIGN: Amy Hansen, Daniel Stewart

Other Titles Available
from Michigan Writers Cooperative Press

The Grace of the Eye by Michael Callaghan
Trouble With Faces by Trinna Frever
Box of Echoes by Todd Mercer
Beyond the Reach of Imagination by Duncan Spratt Moran
The Grass Impossibly by Holly Wren Spaulding
The Chocolatier Speaks of his Wife by Catherine Turnbull
Dangerous Exuberance by Leigh Fairey
Point of Sand by Jaimien Delp
Hard Winter, First Thaw by Jenny Robertson
Friday Nights the Whole Town Goes to the Basketball Game by Teresa J. Scollon
Seasons for Growing by Sarah Baughman
Forking the Swift by Jennifer Sperry Steinorth
The Rest of Us by John Mauk
Kisses for Laura by Joan Schmeichel
Eat the Apple by Denise Baker
First Risings by Michael Hughes
Fathers and Sons by Bruce L. Makie
Exit Wounds by Jim Crockett
The Solid Living World by Ellen Stone
Bitter Dagaa by Robb Astor
Crime Story by Kris Kuntz
Michaela by Gabriella Burman
Supposing She Dreamed This by Gail Wallace Bozzano
Line and Hook by Kevin Griffin
And Sarah His Wife by Christina Diane Campbell
Proud Flesh by Nancy Parshall
Angel Rides a Bike by Margaret Fedder
Ink by Kathleen Pfeiffer
What Will You Teach Her? by Megan Klco Kellner
The Mountain Ash by Kathleen Rabbers
This Blue Earth by Sharon Bippus
Upstairs, Listening by Melida LePere
Twinkies by Kathleen Quigley
The Sound a Car Door Makes by Natalie Tomlin

Michigan
WRITERS

www.ingramcontent.com/pod-product-compliance
Lightning Source LLC
Chambersburg PA
CBHW030141100526
44592CB00011B/1000